High Praise
for
Just Fine

This book provides millions of Americans with the opportunity to truly understand how to maintain quality of life on a day-to-day basis despite a chronic illness or condition. The combination of text and picture tells a complete story from a fresh perspective. Interesting and compelling! I couldn't put it down.   —Gary Collins, actor and talk show host

By juxtaposing compelling human stories and stylish photographs, *Just Fine* proves that visual cues do not give a full picture of disability. Anyone who doesn't believe illness can trick the eye must read this book. The interviews are informative, comprehensive, and surprisingly uplifting.
—Peggy Munson, editor of
Stricken: Voices from the Hidden Epidemic
of Chronic Fatigue Syndrome

Finally a book to hand to patients in which they will recognize themselves and find both practical advice and profound inspiration. Sveilich has brought concealed disorders out of the closet.   —Joan Klagsbrun, Ph.D., psychologist,
professor and director of Wellspring Center,
a center for people with life-changing illness.

We all want to project a healthy visage to the world, but a very strange thing happens when chronic hidden pain wears down our insides without necessarily manifesting itself on the outside. Some of us pretend to be our outsides, and often that leads to despair. Some of us may feel we have to justify our illness, our appearance, our emotional balance and that can lead to bitterness. Carol Sveilich has given our insides a voice and a face, mediums of expression we may have suppressed. She has, therefore, given us hope.
—Laurel Doud, author of *This Body*

Just Fine casts off the cloak of invisibility that surrounds so many chronic conditions. With insight and compassion, it navigates the thoroughfares and byways of the world of concealed illness. This book will be as helpful to those who recognize themselves in its pages as it will be fascinating and moving to those fortunate enough to count themselves strangers to this world.
—Steven Epstein, Ph.D., Medical Sociologist and author of
Impure Science: AIDS, Activism, and the Politics of Knowledge

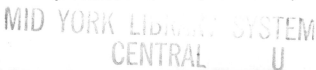

High Praise

for

Just Fine

As one who has lived with a chronic illness most of my life, I find *Just Fine* is a hopeful, useful, easy to read book that comforts and enlightens the reader. If someone you care about lives with a chronic disorder, get them (and their physician) this book. —Mary Ann Mobley, former Miss America, actress, documentary filmmaker

Carol Sveilich took a unique concept and turned it into a masterpiece that clearly communicates the special challenges of those with concealed disorders. *Just Fine* explores the courage that must be manifested and utilized on a daily basis. Inspiring and enlightening!—Pamela Meistrell, Executive Director, Crohn's and Colitis Foundation of America, Greater San Diego and Desert Area Chapters

The *Just Fine* reader will gain an understanding of and empathy for the individual afflicted by concealed chronic illness or pain. For a family or friend of someone affected with a concealed illness, this book will be a real eye-opener. The incorporation of actual people with their photographs and stories makes the information real and conveys the impact of the illness on the individual. —Dr. Terry Cronan, Ph.D., Professor of Psychology, Behavioral Medicine

In *Just Fine: Unmasking Concealed Chronic Illness and Pain,* Carol Sveilich exposes the often hidden world of pain, and the calm, yet heroic way in which people cope. —Hugh Mehan, Ph.D., Professor of Sociology and author of several books in his field

Carol Sveilich has crafted a truly compelling look at chronic illness from the perspective of the patient. Readers will see portraits of courage in these pages, and they will gain both hope and inspiration. *Just Fine* offers a fascinating glimpse at people who struggle with chronic illness every day, yet strive to appear healthy, or whose very illness belies its seriousness by not affecting outward appearance. I don't believe there is another book out there that so perfectly captures this amazing struggle.

—Erica Orloff,
Crohn's disease patient and author

Just Fine